Love Your Diet

Calorie Counter

Maximum Calories

The Goldilocks Paradigm

K.J.R. Alexander

Credits

All amounts are extrapolated for different measurements using
the standardized US Department of Agriculture Nutrient Database:

http://www.nal.usda.gov/fnic/foodcomp/

USDA National Nutrient Database for Standard Reference
Release 22 (2009)

CONTENTS

Introduction

The Love Your Diet *Calorie Counter* is designed to accompany the Love Your Diet books *Light Fantastic* and *Calories & Real Foods.* These books explain the diet in detail and reading one of them is necessary for full understanding of the dynamics. Charts, tables and menus are included. However, a summary of the diet basics is also included here for reference.

The calorie counter is divided into two parts: calories for the basic good foods to eat on the diet and calories for the foods not to eat – fast foods and the LTN, or Little-To-No foods, as discussed in the books. This helps guide food selection. Following is basic information needed to help guide your diet and count calories.

Maximum Calories: The Goldilocks Paradigm

Not too much and not too little. This is the Goldilocks Paradigm (*pair' a dime*), a pattern or model of thought, used by physicists in the study of the universe. The idea is that everything is balanced and in harmony, as, for example, the stronger and weaker forces in gravity. Not too much and not too little keeps everything just right. Extremes are not the essence. The real essence is somewhere in-between.

Remember, Goldilocks, in the Three Bears' house, checks the chairs, beds, and bowls of porridge belonging to Papa Bear, Mama Bear and Baby Bear. She finds Papa and Mama Bear's too much and too little, but Baby Bear's, for her, are just right! Goldilocks can help! Not too much and not too little, but just right, is a model for the universe. It is also a model to use for your calories for healthy effective dieting.

If you are serious about losing excess weight, the question is not whether you need to count calories. The question is how can you **not** count calories and succeed in the long run. If you don't count calories, you are using someone else's lopsided starvation diet. Calorie counting is the only sane way to mathematically keep track of what you are eating with freedom, choice, and nutrition. Meanwhile, you learn the calorie values of different foods and learn how to read food labels, so necessary in the modern food culture. However, diets that restrict calories to severe limits are not the answer either. Nutritionally unbalanced and severely restricted diets are counterproductive and even dangerous to health. After losing the excess fat, you will not need to count calories.

How Many Calories Do You Need Each Day?

Not too much and not too little, but just right. This is the amount of food you can eat and still lose weight without hunger while following the plan. This is based on the amount of food you are currently eating. Therefore, to count calories for Love Your Diet, you first calculate how many calories you are eating now and set this as your daily upper limit in calories. Some days you will be more hungry and go a little over the target amount. Other days, you will eat less. As you lose weight, your target number for calories also declines. *The effect is that the body naturally relaxes its storage of fat as you replace bad foods with the good foods that are metabolized efficiently.*

How many calories are you now eating to support you current weight? To calculate this amount, simply multiply your current weight by 12, an energy factor selected in Love Your Diet for a sedentary type lifestyle such as sitting at computers or desks and moderate walking. To calculate total calories with the energy factor:

Your current weight x 12 = Your total daily calories.

If you are too hungry, try a 15 factor. The factor is flexible and variable among individuals. What matters is whether you are losing excess fat at the rate of two to five pounds or more per week. This is a real and gentle fat melt and not just water weight as on other diets.

For example, if you weigh 185 pounds, the amount at the 12 factor will be 185 x 12 = 2220 calories, your upper calorie limit for the day. As you eat your own target calories of the good foods guided by the calorie counter, your body automatically reduces fat. Without hunger! As you lose weight, say every five to ten pounds, you will reduce your upper limit in calories. The beauty of this diet is that you will lose weight while eating within 10 pounds of your upper range in calories, *if you are eating the right foods*. You have to severely restrict calories to lose weight *eating the wrong foods*, in turn causing tormenting hunger pains and a body ready to fight back and regain all the fat. Eating good foods but *still eating* the bad foods will also result in no fat loss. The reason is that the good foods can be metabolized and the bad foods "stick to the body" in excess fat. All calories are not equal with today's industrialized foods! This is explained fully in the books.

By putting calories per pound with the 12 factor to work for yourself, you can compare each day's calorie intake and weight to see how calories and weight interact. *You can see how your body, when you are eating the natural carbohydrate metabolizer foods, asks with hunger, which you immediately satisfy, for calories just under those required to maintain overweight, with the effect of reducing fat.* If you find you are too hungry, or eating more calories than the amount calculated at the 12 factor, again, you can try a little higher factor, such as 15. The factor is flexible as long as you are losing weight. However, at first, begin the 12 factor as a good starting point.

What Should You Weigh?

Are you overweight? How much do you have to lose to be within a healthy to moderate weight range for your height? Measuring BMI or Body Mass Index is one way to determine where you stand. BMI indicates how much excess fat is on your body. Here is a table that gives height, weight, and BMI. While these amounts are general averages, they are good indicators of healthy weight range. If your weight is not listed due to space limitations, such as 5'8" at 192, which is obese at 197, your category would be in the overweight range bordering on obese. You can also calculate your own BMI online.

BMI	19	20	21	22	23	24	25	26	27	28	29	30	31	32	33	34	35

Height & Weight in Pounds

	Healthy Weight						Overweight					Obese					
4'10"	91	96	100	105	110	115	119	124	129	134	138	143	148	153	158	162	167
4'11"	94	99	104	109	114	119	124	128	133	138	143	148	153	158	163	168	173
5'	97	102	107	112	118	123	128	133	138	143	148	153	158	163	158	174	179
5'1"	100	106	111	116	122	127	132	137	143	148	153	158	164	169	174	180	185
5'2"	104	109	115	120	126	131	136	142	147	153	158	164	169	175	180	186	191
5'3"	107	113	118	124	130	135	141	146	152	158	163	169	175	180	186	191	197
5'4"	110	116	122	128	134	140	145	151	157	163	169	174	180	186	192	197	204
5'5"	114	120	126	132	138	144	150	156	162	168	174	180	186	192	198	204	210
5'6"	118	124	130	136	142	148	155	161	167	173	179	186	192	198	204	210	216
5'7"	121	127	134	140	146	153	159	166	172	178	185	191	198	204	211	217	223
5'8"	125	131	138	144	151	158	164	171	177	184	190	197	203	210	216	223	230
5'9"	128	135	142	149	155	162	169	176	182	189	196	203	209	216	223	230	236
5'10"	132	139	146	153	160	167	174	181	188	195	202	209	216	222	229	236	243
5'11"	136	143	150	157	165	172	179	186	193	200	208	215	222	229	236	243	250
6'	140	147	154	162	169	177	184	191	199	206	213	221	228	235	242	250	258
6'1"	144	151	159	166	174	182	189	197	204	212	219	227	235	242	250	257	265
6'2"	148	155	163	171	179	186	194	202	210	218	225	233	241	249	256	264	272
6'3"	152	160	168	176	184	192	200	208	216	224	232	240	248	256	264	272	279

Source: Evidence Report of Clinical Guidelines on the Identification, Evaluation, and Treatment of Overweight and Obesity in Adults, 1998. NIH/National Heart, Lung, and Blood Institute (NHLB). Posted at USDA.

Following are two more charts to help you get an idea of how your weight compares.

AVERAGE WEIGHTS AND OVERWEIGHTS FOR MEN AND WOMEN

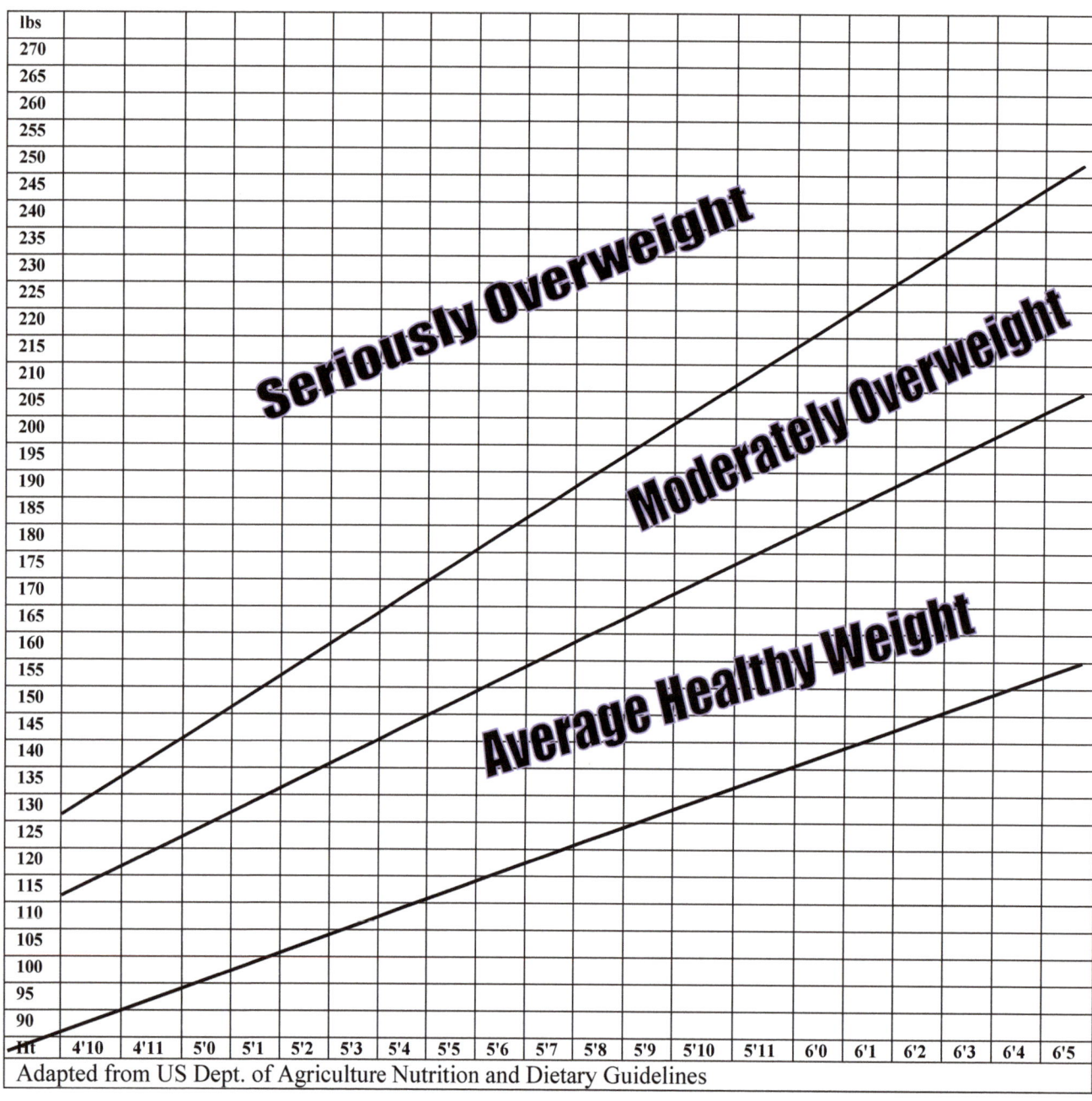

Adapted from US Dept. of Agriculture Nutrition and Dietary Guidelines

Average Healthy Weights for Men and Women by Height and Bone Structure

Women

Average Weights by Height and Bone Structure
without shoes or clothes

	Small	Medium	Large
5'11"	135 to 148	145 to 159	155 to 176
5'10	132 to 145	142 to 156	152 to 172
5'9"	129 to 142	139 to 153	149 to 170
5'8"	126 to 139	136 to 150	146 to 167
5'7"	123 to 136	133 to 147	143 to 163
5'6"	120 to 133	130 to 144	140 to 159
5'5"	117 to 130	127 to 141	137 to 155
5'4"	114 to 127	124 to 138	134 to 151
5'3"	111 to 124	121 to 135	131 to 147
5'2"	108 to 121	118 to 132	128 to 143
5'1"	105 to 118	115 to 129	125 to 140
5'0"	103 to 115	112 to 126	122 to 137
4'11"	101 to 112	110 to 123	119 to 134
4'10"	100 to 110	108 to 120	117 to 131
4'9"	99 to 108	106 to 118	115 to 128

To Determine Bone Structure:

Grasp wrist with opposite hand.
Fingers overlap: Small bone structure
Fingers barely touch: Medium bone structure
Fingers separated: Large bone structure

Men

Average Weights by Height and Bone Structure
without shoes or clothes

	Small	Medium	Large
6'3"	157 to 172	167 to 182	176 to 202
6'2"	153 to 167	163 to 177	171 to 197
6'1"	150 to 163	159 to 173	167 to 192
6'0	147 to 159	155 to 169	163 to 187
5'11"	144 to 155	152 to 165	159 to 183
5'10	141 to 152	149 to 161	156 to 179
5'9"	139 to 149	146 to 158	153 to 175
5'8"	137 to 146	143 to 155	150 to 171
5'7"	135 to 143	140 to 152	147 to 167
5'6"	133 to 140	137 to 149	144 to 163
5'5"	131 to 137	134 to 146	141 to 159
5'4"	129 to 135	132 to 143	139 to 155
5'3"	127 to 133	130 to 140	137 to 151
5'2"	125 to 131	128 to 138	135 to 148
5'1"	123 to 129	126 to 136	133 to 145

Metropolitan Life Insurance Tables, 1983

Weigh Yourself Every Day
Your *Daily Weight and Calorie Journal*

A dieter needs more direction and guidance than just foregoing certain foods in order to stay focused on the diet. The temptation to eat is everywhere in the food environment. It's just too easy to stray once, twice, and thrice, then back to the old eating habits. This is why a *Daily Weight and Calorie Journal* you write yourself is needed. You are able to see the immediate effects of certain foods. You can see on paper the record of what you have eaten and what you weigh each day.

You need to weigh yourself each morning before eating or drinking, without clothes or in the same type clothes each day. You will then list the foods you eat each day and total the calories at the end of the day. You can also write down as many or as few of your thoughts of the day as you wish, your feelings and actions, and what is occurring in your life. You are then more aware of stress and frustration and their possible influences on your eating habits. When you feel good, you can also make note. Your *Daily Weight and Calorie Journal* is a personal part of the adventure into yourself as you lose weight. A piece of paper and pencil will do as will any format you choose, but keep each day's record so you can refer back to it and see progress. For more explanation, see Chapter 8, *Maximum Calories* in Love Your Diet's *Light Fantastic*.

DIET PLAN SUMMARY

Following is a highly-condensed version of Love Your Diet *Light Fantastic*. For more understanding, you need to read the whole book. Love Your Diet is more than calorie counting and is a lot about *how* to choose the right foods. The result is a diet of freedom with lots of choices in foods. However, the following guide is an excellent way to begin to apply your calorie counting.

Stop Starch & Sugar Addiction

If you are overweight, you are eating foods that cause the weight gain. These are manufactured starch and sugar type foods. These foods are addictive and contribute to the constant felt need to eat more and too much. These are the foods on grocery shelves, packaged and full of ingredients that stifle metabolism. It is not enough to only give up foods with gluten, or with corn syrup or sugar, or fat, or certain chemicals, or whatever. These are the foods manufactured for profit rather than for healthy metabolism. To begin the weight loss and to eat comfortably on the diet, you need to give up manufactured, industrialized starch and sugar. Starch and sugar foods are carbohydrate foods. But you do not have to give up carbohydrates. You need only replace the *highly-processed* carbohydrates with *natural* carbohydrates. By following the Love Your Diet *Calorie Counter* as a guide and avoiding the Fast Food Fat and LTN (Little-to-No) Foods, you will be selecting the right foods that are compatible with your natural metabolism. Be sure to eat a variety of foods each day with lots of fruits and vegetables to maintain the balance needed for metabolic energies.

Natural Carbohydrates

You do not have to give up the body's need for carbohydrate foods. You need only to replace the manufactured foods with the natural, real carbohydrates your body can metabolize. This includes a rich cornucopia of lush fruits, vegetables, natural sweets such as honey and raw sugar, and heavy duty natural carbs such as potatoes, rice, beans, and even pasta and bread. This is shown in the calorie counters. Included are the **S** or Sometimes foods and the **LTN** Foods, while losing weight. Bread needs to be all-natural and bakery fresh without added preservatives. See a table of grain products from least to most fattening in *Light Fantastic* or the *Aphrodite Bread and Wine Diet*.

High Protein

Protein is very important to the body. Protein is needed to repair, replace, and build all the cells in the body including muscle, organs, skin, and hair. Adequate protein also helps curb hunger and prevent fatigue while dieting. It also helps maintain skin tone and the skin's ability to "tighten up" and shrink with weight loss. Of the three food categories of carbohydrates, proteins, and fats, protein is the most difficult category to maintain in adequate amounts during dieting. Needed are the foods which supply the EAAs or Essential Amino Acids. (Amino acids are protein.) The body needs daily EAAs in the diet. These are the proteins the body cannot manufacture on its own and must be supplied every day by the diet. To ensure excellent metabolic material, adequate protein is especially needed by the dieter. Foods that contain EAAs, or complete protein are dairy products and meat products such as fish, shellfish, poultry, pork, and beef. Dairy products include milk, yogurt, cottage cheese, and cheese. Eggs also supply complete protein and are very nutritious. Soybean products are the only plant food classified as a complete protein. However, all foods, even fruits and vegetables, have little protein players that contribute to protein synthesis. For this reason, protein amounts are listed in the calorie counters. *For calculating total protein however, you need to count only the EAA foods. These are shown in the last column in the calorie counters in red and show the amount of protein for Column B amounts.*

How much protein do you need each day?

This amount is much higher than most of us eat, especially while dieting. The National Academy of Sciences fixes the amount at half your normal weight. This means your *target* weight, not your overweight. For example, your normal target healthy weight is 160 pounds. This means you should eat half that amount in protein grams or around 80 grams of protein. You may eat more or less than this amount, but this is the target amount. Again, this is calculated using the EAA foods. While dieting, it is especially important to get a good start on the day with a protein breakfast. By contributing to protein needs throughout the day, you are providing adequate metabolic material to burn that excess fat and prevent hunger and fatigue. Love Your Diet structures protein intake throughout the day as shown next in the Daily Menu Model.

No Hunger

Maximum Calories

This is described above in the 12 factor calculation and is accomplished using the calorie charts.

Eat When Hungry

Three levels of hunger are identified in *Love Your Diet*.

Hunger Level 1

This is the first twinges of hunger, the signal that you need to eat soon. Level 1 Hunger can be forgotten for small amounts of time.

Hunger Level 2

This is constant feelings of hunger that do not go away. The body signals the need for food.

Hunger Level 3

This is the level of hunger when the body feels it is starving and must have food immediately! Of course, you know it has fat stores to use and is not starving. However this is a survival mechanism by the body. The body is not programmed to endure hunger but interprets Level 3 Hunger as danger of starvation. Willpower can hold up to Level 3 Hunger only so long and then the strongest-willed gives in to the fattest food he or she can find.

On Love Your Diet, Hunger Level 3 is to be avoided! *You are to eat at Level 1 Hunger.* This assures the body that food is available and it is safe to burn excess fat. Again, this is more completely explained in the book, Love Your Diet *Light Fantastic* or *Calories & Real Foods,* which also include starter menus.

To repeat, as you eat to prevent hunger, but **without highly processed starch and sugar products**, you will see how your body, *on its own*, decreases calorie demand. You immediately feel better and have more energy. The feeling of well-being is so great, you will gladly continue your diet. After all, you are not starving, you are not hungry, and you are replacing empty fat-producing calories with the nutritious food your body appreciates. The body, rather than being signaled to store fat for famine, now feels comfortable with the abundance of nutritious more easily metabolized food such as dairy products, meat, fruits, and vegetables. The body adapts for the "good times" of abundant food supply, close to the land, with good weather and water. Again, this is explained more in the books *Light Fantastic* and *Calories & Real Foods.*

For now, prepare to weigh yourself every morning and count your daily calories determined by the 12 factor calculation. Eat natural, fresh, real foods indicated in the calorie counters. The excess fat will melt away while you are experiencing a satisfying gourmet diet!

DAILY MENU MODEL
Breakfast
15 to 20 grams protein

As dairy is the most compatible with breakfast, this includes milk or dairy products such as yogurt, cottage cheese, and eggs. Kefir is also a highly nutritious filling drink you may want to try if you like buttermilk. You may also use commercial high protein drinks. Read the labels. Include fresh, raw fruit, such as blueberries, apricots, peaches, apples, etc.

Hunger Level 1 Snacks, Morning
8 to 10 grams protein

Hunger level snacks include lowfat dairy foods such as yogurt or cottage cheese and fresh, raw juicy fruit such as cherries and strawberries. High protein drinks may also be used. Eat as much as wanted. Do not choose yogurt packed with extra sugar. Choose the low sugar or artificially sweetened kind around 100 calories. You can also mix all-natural yogurt with no-sugar-added with 1 or 2 tablespoons of the artificially-sweetened and flavored variety, a mixture called LYD or Love Your Diet Yogurt.

Lunch
20+ grams protein
Chicken or fish and raw vegetables and/or raw, fresh fruit.

Hunger Level 1 Snacks, Afternoon
8 to 10 grams protein
Same as morning.

Before Dinner, while preparing food
Raw, fresh vegetables and fruit. Table wine if wanted.

Dinner
20+ grams protein
Meat type food (fish, poultry, beef), heavy duty carb such as potato, rice, or beans, and steamed fresh vegetable with sour cream. Table wine if wanted.

Dessert
Fresh raw fruit with chocolate sauce, honey, raw sugar, no-sugar-added ice cream or cream. Example: banana split with ice cream, chocolate sauce, and peanuts. 70% or more cacao chocolate bar is also good.

After Dinner Hunger Snack
Repeat dessert or choose from nibblers such as nuts, dried fruit, seeds.

Anytime Beverages
These include water, tea, coffee, and moderate intake of diet soda. To flavor tea or coffee, use natural raw sugar or honey and real cream, milk, or half and half and not the artificial creamers. To flavor water, use a tablespoon of all natural, no-sugar-added condensed fruit juice such as cranberry or a fresh lemon.

Again, menus and food lists are available in *Light Fantastic* and *Calories & Real Foods*.

Calorie Counters

The two Love Your Diet Calorie Counters are designed for easy use. Here's how to read the calorie counters. The first amount in **Column A**, gives a small portion measure followed in the next column by the calories, which can be multiplied times the amount eaten. Or as an option, the second amount in **Column B** gives the amount of an average serving and the total calories in the following column. The last column is the **Protein Column** showing protein for the measure in Column B. All protein is shown for interest and to indicate all the protein players. As stated earlier, the amount for complete protein foods, Essential Amino Acids or EAAs, are the only proteins to be counted for your daily protein intake and are listed in red.

The first part of the calorie counter is the Love Your Diet *Calorie Counter* specifically designed for the diet. The amounts are rounded to the nearest 5 to help daily calculations. This guides food choices that are harmonious to the body's need for nutrition and therefore metabolism. The second part lists calories for *Fast Foods and LTN Foods*, those to avoid while reducing excess fat. These amounts are not rounded to the nearest 5.

Here are the supplies you need for counting calories:

Weight scale for weighing yourself each morning before eating or drinking
Food scale for weighing food in serving sizes in ounces up to at least a pound
Individual measuring cups 2 C, 1 C, ½ C, ¼ C (C= Cup)
1 Tablespoon measure T or tablespoon in the diet
1 teaspoon measure tsp or teaspoon in the diet
Calculator
This Love Your Diet Calorie Counter
Your Daily Weight and Calorie Journal you write

Love Your Diet
Calorie Counter

FOODS TO EAT

Measurements and Abbreviations

The following list accompanies your Calorie Counter with explanation of abbreviations and measurements as well as notes about the lists.

---

lb = pound (16 oz)   oz = ounce   C = cup (8 oz)

T = Tablespoon   t or tsp = teaspoon   g = grams

1/4 C = 2 oz   1/2 C = 4 oz   3/4 C = 6 oz   1C = 8 oz

1/ 4 C = 4T   1/2 C = 8T   3/4 C = 12T   1C = 16T   1T = 3 tsp

1 oz = 28.35 grams   3.5 oz = 100 grams   1 lb = 16 oz or 453.6 grams
1 gal = 4 quarts = 3.786 liters = 378 milliliters(ml)   1 quart = 4 C = 2 pints = 946 liter = .946 ml   1C = 30 ml

---

Please note: The calorie amounts are rounded to the nearest 5 for easier calculation. This accounts for differences in exact Column A and Column B amounts.
Amounts in Fast Foods and LTN Foods are not rounded.

Use Calorie Counter amounts to easily calculate calories for servings of different sizes.
Add cooking calories such as cooking oil to cooked food.
Packaged foods: Check labels for calories.
LTN = Little-to-No Intake Foods   S = Sometimes (may be eaten sometimes on diet)
***Protein grams are for B serving amounts.* Less than .5 gram protein = <.5**
EAA, Essential Amino Acid, proteins listed in red.

Food	Type	A Calories		B Calories		B Protein Grams EAA
A						
alfalfa sprouts	raw	**1/2 C**	5	**1 C**	10	1
almonds, see nuts, almonds						
apple	raw, unpeeled	**1 oz**	15	**5 oz**	80	<.5
apple	raw, diced, chopped	**1/4 C**	15	**1 C**	65	<.5
apple butter	spread	**1 T**	30	**2 T**	60	<.5
apple juice, canned or bottled	unsweetened	**1/2 C**	60	**1 C**	120	<.5
applesauce	canned, unsweetened	**1/2 C**	50	**1 C**	105	<.5
apricot	raw	**1 apricot**	20	**1/2C halves**	75	2
apricot, dried	unsweetened, halves	**1/2 C**	155	**1 C**	310	4
artichokes	raw	**1 oz**	15	**1 med**	60	4
artichokes, hearts	cooked	**1/2 C**	40	**1 C**	80	6
asparagus	cooked	**1/2 C**	10	**1 C**	20	4
avocado	peeled, pitted	**1 oz**	45	**7 oz**	315	4
avocado	peeled, sliced	**1/2 C**	115	**1 C**	235	3
B						
bacon, canadian style LTN	cured, cooked	**1 oz**	50	**2 sl**	90	**12**
bacon, pork, cured LTN	pan fried	**1 oz**	155	**1 sl**	45	**3**
bamboo shoots	canned, drained	**1/2 C**	10	**1 C**	25	2
banana	raw	**1 oz**	25	**5 oz**	125	2
bean sprouts, mung	raw	**1/2 C**	15	**1 C**	30	3
bean sprouts, soybean	raw	**1/2 C**	45	**1 C**	90	9
beans, black	cooked	**1/2 C**	115	**1 C**	230	15
beans, garbanzo or chickpeas	cooked	**1/2 C**	140	**1 C**	270	13
beans, great northern	cooked	**1/2 C**	105	**1 C**	210	15

beans, lentils	cooked	**1/2 C**	115	**1 C**	230	18
beans, lima	cooked	**1/2 C**	110	**1 C**	215	15
beans, pea, navy	cooked	**1/2 C**	130	**1 C**	260	15
beans, pinto	cooked	**1/2 C**	125	**1 C**	245	15
beans, red kidney	cooked	**1/2 C**	110	**1 C**	225	15
beans, snap, green, yellow	raw, cooked	**1/2 C**	25	**1 C**	45	2
beans, soy	dry, cooked	**1/2 C**	150	**1 C**	300	29
Beef						
beef, bottom round, rump roast	cooked, lean only	**1 oz**	55	**4 oz**	220	31
beef, bottom round, steak	raw, lean only	**1 oz**	45	**4 oz**	180	24
beef, chuck, arm roast	cooked, lean only	**1 oz**	55	**4 oz**	220	38
beef, chuck, blade roast	cooked, lean only	**1 oz**	65	**4 oz**	260	35
beef, corned	cooked	**1 oz**	70	**4 oz**	280	21
beef, eye of round	raw	**1 oz**	40	**4 oz**	160	25
beef, eye of round	roasted	**1 oz**	45	**4 oz**	180	33
beef, flank steak	raw	**1 oz**	40	**4 oz**	160	24
beef, flank steak	cooked	**1 oz**	55	**4 oz**	220	32
beef, ground, 75% lean	raw	**1 oz**	80	**4 oz**	320	17
beef, ground, 75% lean	cooked	**1 oz**	70	**4 oz**	280	27
beef, ground, 80% lean	raw	**1 oz**	70	**4 oz**	280	19
beef, ground, 80% lean	cooked	**1 oz**	70	**4 oz**	280	27
beef, ground, 90% lean	raw	**1 oz**	50	**4 oz**	200	23
beef, ground, 90% lean	cooked	**1 oz**	60	**4 oz**	240	29
beef, ground, 95% lean	raw	**1 oz**	40	**4 oz**	160	24
beef, ground, 95% lean	cooked	**1 oz**	45	**4 oz**	180	29
beef, heart	raw	**1 oz**	30	**4 oz**	120	19
beef, kidney	raw	**1 oz**	35	**4 oz**	140	17
beef, liver	raw	**1 oz**	40	**4 oz**	160	23
beef, liver	fried	**1 oz**	50	**4 oz**	200	30

beef, porterhouse steak	raw, 1/4" fat	**1 oz**	65	**4 oz**	260	**22**
beef, porterhouse steak	broiled, lean only	**1 oz**	60	**4 oz**	240	**31**
beef, rib eye steak	broiled, lean only	**1 oz**	60	**4 oz**	240	**30**
beef, rib roast	roasted, lean only	**1 oz**	60	**4 oz**	240	**30**
beef, round tip roast	cooked, lean only	**1 oz**	55	**4 oz**	260	**31**
beef, round, top round	raw, lean only	**1 oz**	40	**4 oz**	160	**26**
beef, round, top round	cooked, lean only	**1 oz**	55	**4 oz**	220	**36**
beef, sirloin, top sirloin	raw, lean only	**1 oz**	35	**4 oz**	140	**25**
beef, sirloin, top sirloin	cooked, lean only	**1 oz**	50	**4 oz**	200	**35**
beef, sirloin, tri tip	raw	**1 oz**	45	**4 oz**	180	**23**
beef, sirloin, tri tip	roasted	**1 oz**	60	**4 oz**	240	**29**
beef, t bone steak	raw, 1/4" fat	**1 oz**	45	**4 oz**	180	**24**
beef, t bone steak	broiled, lean only	**1 oz**	60	**4 oz**	240	**31**
beef, tenderloin	raw, 1/8" fat trim	**1 oz**	45	**4 oz**	180	**25**
beef, tenderloin	broiled, 1/8" fat trim	**1 oz**	60	**4 oz**	240	**33**
beer, 12 oz	regular	**1 oz**	13	**12 oz**	155	2
beer, 12 oz	light	**1 oz**	9	**12 oz**	105	1
beer, 16 oz	regular	**1 oz**	13	**16 oz**	210	2
beer, 16 oz	light	**1 oz**	9	**16 oz**	145	1
beet greens	cooked	**1/2 C**	15	**1 C**	30	4
beets	cooked, slices	**1/2 C**	40	**1 C**	75	3
bison, ground (buffalo)	cooked, patty	**1 oz**	65	**4 oz**	260	**27**
black eyed peas	cooked	**1/2 C**	90	**1 C**	180	7
blackberries	raw	**1/2 C**	30	**1 C**	60	2
blueberries	raw	**1/2 C**	40	**1 C**	85	1
bok choy, Chinese cabbage	cooked, sliced	**1/2 C**	10	**1 C**	20	3
boysenberries	frozen, unsweetened	**1 /2 C**	30	**1 C**	60	1
brazil nuts, see nuts						
bread, buns, hamb, hot dog LTN	enriched	**1 avg**	120	**1 avg**	120	3

bread, corn bread S	from recipe 2% milk	1 oz	75	2 oz	150	4
bread, French or sourdough S	loaf, bakery	1 oz	78	2 oz	155	5
bread, Indian fry S	Navajo	1 oz	94	2 oz	188	4
bread, Italian S	enriched, loaf, bakery	1 oz	77	2 oz	155	5
bread, kneel down S	Navajo	1 oz	55	2 oz	110	2
bread, mixed grain LTN	sliced, shelf	1 oz	70	26 g sl	65	3
bread, pita S	4" diameter	1 oz	80	1 4" pita	80	3
bread, pumpernickel S	loaf	1 oz	70	2 oz	140	5
bread, raisin LTN	sliced, shelf	1 oz	78	26 g sl	70	2
bread, rye S	American, sliced	1 oz	75	32 g sl	85	3
bread, wheat LTN	sliced, shelf	1 oz	70	28 g sl	70	3
bread, white, enriched LTN	sliced, shelf	1oz	75	25 g sl	65	2
bread, white, enriched S	homebaked 2% milk	1 oz	80	2 oz	160	4
bread, white S	homebkd nonfat milk	1 oz	78	2 oz	160	4
breakfast bars	oats, raisins, coconut	1 oz	130	43 g bar	200	8
brewers yeast	flakes/supplement	1 T	25	2 T	50	6
broccoli	cooked, chopped	1/2 C	30	1 C	60	4
broccoli	raw, chopped	1/2 C	15	1 C	30	3
broccoli spear	cooked, 5" long spear	1 spear	10	5" stalk	50	3
broccoli, flower cluster	raw	1 floweret	5	1 C	20	2
brussels sprouts	cooked	1/2 C	30	1 C	60	4
bulgar	cooked	1/2 C	75	1 C	150	6
butter	spread	1 tsp	35	1 T	100	<.5

C

cabbage, Chinese	cooked, sliced	1/2 C	10	1 C	20	3
cabbage, common varieties	raw, shredded	1/2 C	10	1 C	20	<1
cabbage, common varieties	cooked	1/2 C	15	1 C	30	2
cabbage, red	raw, shredded	1/2 C	10	1 C	20	1

cabbage, savoy	raw, sliced	1/2 C	10	1 C	20	2
cantaloupe	raw, 5" diam. melon	1/2 melon	95	1 melon	190	1
cantaloupe	raw, cubes	1/2 C	55	1 C	110	1
carrot, baby	raw	1 med	5	4 med	20	<.5
carrots	raw, grated	1 oz	12	1 C	50	1
carrots	cooked	1/2 C	35	1 C	70	1
casaba melon	raw	1/10th avg	40	1 melon	380	2
cashews, see nuts						
catsup	tomato	1 T	15	2 T	30	<1
cauliflower	raw, floweret	1	5	1 C	25	2
cauliflower	cooked	1/2 C	15	1 C	30	2
caviar	red, black	1 T	40	3 T	120	12
celery	raw	1 stalk	5	1 C	20	1
celery	cooked	1/2 C	15	1 C	30	1
cereal, corn grits, white, yellow	dry, uncooked	1/4 C	145	1/2 C	290	7
cereal, corn grits, white, yellow	cooked	1/2 C	70	1 C	145	3
cereal, cream of rice	dry, uncooked	1/4 C	160	1/2 C	320	5
cereal, cream of rice	cooked	1/2 C	65	1 C	125	2
cereal, oats, rolled	dry, uncooked	1/4 C	75	1/2 C	155	6
cereal, oats, rolled	cooked	1/2 C	70	1 C	145	6
cereal, whole wheat natural	dry, uncooked	1/4 C	80	1/2 C	160	5
cereal, whole wheat natural	cooked	1/2 C	80	1 C	160	5
champagne	all	1 oz	25	4 oz	100	<.5
chard, Swiss	raw or cooked	1/2 C	15	1 C	25	3
cheese, American	sliced	1 oz	105	2 oz	210	14
cheese, average	grated	1 T	25	2 oz	50	4
cheese, average	sliced	1 oz	100	2 oz	200	14
cheese, brie	sliced	1 oz	95	2 oz	190	12
cheese, camembert	sliced	1 oz	85	2 oz	170	12

cheese, cheddar	grated	**1 T**	30	**2 T**	60	3
cheese, cheddar	sliced	**1 oz**	115	**2 oz**	230	14
cheese, colby	sliced	**1 oz**	110	**2 oz**	220	14
cheese, cream cheese	spread	**1 oz**	105	**2 oz**	210	4
cheese, edam	sliced	**1 oz**	100	**2 oz**	200	15
cheese, feta	sliced	**1 oz**	75	**2 oz**	150	8
cheese, gouda	sliced	**1 oz**	100	**2 oz**	200	14
cheese, monterey	sliced	**1 oz**	105	**2 oz**	210	14
cheese, mozzarella	sliced	**1 oz**	80	**2 oz**	160	12
cheese, muenster	sliced	**1 oz**	105	**2 oz**	210	14
cheese, parmesan	grated	**1 T**	25	**2 T**	50	4
cheese, parmesan	cubed	**1 oz**	110	**1 oz**	110	10
cheese, provolone	sliced	**1 oz**	100	**2 oz**	200	15
cheese, Swiss	sliced	**1 oz**	105	**2 oz**	210	15
cherries	raw, sweet	**1/2 C**	40	**1 C**	80	2

Chicken

Amounts do not include bone weight. Weigh bone after eating and subtract from total weight.

chicken, breast, meat & skin	batter dipped, fried	**1 oz**	75	**4 oz**	300	28
chicken, breast, meat & skin	flour coated, fried	**1 oz**	65	**4 oz**	260	36
chicken, breast, meat & skin	fried	**1 oz**	60	**4 oz**	240	36
chicken, breast, meat & skin	roasted	**1 oz**	55	**4 oz**	220	34
chicken, breast, meat only	fried	**1 oz**	55	**4 oz**	220	38
chicken, breast, meat only	roasted	**1 oz**	45	**4 oz**	180	35
chicken, broiler fryer, meat & skin	batter dipped, fried	**1 oz**	80	**4 oz**	320	26
chicken, broiler fryer, meat & skin	flour coated, fried	**1 oz**	75	**4 oz**	300	32
chicken, broiler fryer, meat & skin	roasted	**1 oz**	70	**4 oz**	280	31
chicken, broiler fryer, meat & skin	fried	**1 oz**	65	**4 oz**	260	32
chicken, broiler fryer, meat only	roasted	**1 oz**	55	**4 oz**	220	33
chicken, broiler fryer, meat only	fried	**1 oz**	60	**4 oz**	240	34

chicken, broiler fryer, meat only	stewed	1/2 C	125	1 C	250	31
chicken, Cornish game hen	roasted, meat & skin	1/2 bird	335	1 whole	670	57
chicken, Cornish game hen	roasted, meat & skin	1 oz	75	4 oz	300	25
chicken, drumstick, meat & skin	flour coated, fried	1 oz	70	4 oz	280	31
chicken, drumstick, meat & skin	fried	1 oz	60	4 oz	240	31
chicken, drumstick, meat & skin	roasted	1 oz	60	4 oz	240	31
chicken, drumstick, meat & skin	batter dipped, fried	1 oz	75	4 oz	300	25
chicken, drumstick, meat only	fried	1 oz	55	4 oz	220	32
chicken, drumstick, meat only	roasted	1 oz	50	4 oz	200	32
chicken, giblets	simmered, diced	1/2 C	115	1 C	230	39
chicken, leg, meat & skin	batter dipped, fried	1 oz	75	4 oz	300	25
chicken, leg, meat & skin	flour coated, fried	1 oz	70	4 oz	280	30
chicken, leg, meat & skin	fried	1 oz	65	4 oz	260	30
chicken, leg, meat & skin	roasted	1 oz	65	4 oz	260	29
chicken, leg, meat only	fried	1 oz	60	4 oz	240	32
chicken, leg, meat only	roasted	1 oz	55	4 oz	220	31
chicken, liver	fried	1 oz	50	4 oz	200	29
chicken, roasting, meat & skin	roasted	1 oz	65	4 oz	260	27
chicken, roasting, meat only	roasted	1 oz	50	4 oz	200	28
chicken, stewing, meat only	stewed, diced	1/2 C	165	1 C	330	43
chicken, thigh, meat & skin	flour coated, fried	1 oz	75	4 oz	300	30
chicken, thigh, meat & skin	fried	1 oz	65	4 oz	260	30
chicken, thigh, meat & skin	roasted	1 oz	70	4 oz	280	28
chicken, thigh, meat & skin	batter dipped, fried	1 oz	80	4 oz	320	25
chicken, thigh, meat only	fried	1 oz	65	4 oz	260	31
chicken, thigh, meat only	roasted	1 oz	60	4 oz	240	30
chicken, thigh, meat & skin	batter dipped, fried	1 oz	80	4 oz	320	25
chicken, thigh, meat only	fried	1 oz	65	4 oz	260	31
chicken, thigh, meat only	roasted	1 oz	60	4 oz	240	30

chicken, wing, meat & skin	batter dipped, fried	1 oz	90	4 oz	360	23
chicken, wing, meat & skin	flour coated, fried	1 oz	90	4 oz	360	30
chicken, wing, meat & skin	fried	1 oz	70	4 oz	280	31
chicken, wing, meat & skin	roasted	1 oz	80	4 oz	320	30
chicken, wing, meat only	fried	1 oz	60	4 oz	240	34
chicken, wing, meat only	roasted	1 oz	60	4 oz	240	34
chives	raw, chopped	1 T	1	3 T	5	<.5
chocolate fudge topping	thick	1 T	65	2 T	135	2
chocolate syrup topping	thin	1 T	55	2 T	110	1
cocktail sauce, seafood	regular	1 T	10	1/4 C	45	1
coconut	raw	1 oz	100	2 oz	200	2
coconut, flaked	dried, sweetened	1 T	20	1 C	350	2
cod liver oil	supplement/Vit A & D	1 tsp	40	1 T	125	0
coffee	brewed plain	6 oz	2	8 oz	2	<.5
coffee, espresso	brewed plain	1 oz	1	2 oz	1	<.5
coleslaw	home prepared	1/2 C	40	1 C	80	2
collards	raw, chopped	1/2 C	10	1 C	20	2
collards	cooked, chopped	1/2 C	25	1 C	50	4
corn	cooked	1 med ear	75	1 C	130	5
corn grits cereal, white, yellow	dry, uncooked	1/4 C	145	1/2 C	290	7
corn grits cereal, white, yellow	cooked	1/2 C	70	1 C	145	3
cornish game hen	roasted, meat & skin	1/2 bird	335	1 whole	670	57
cornish game hen	roasted, meat & skin	1 oz	75	4 oz	300	25
cornmeal, white or yellow	wholegrain	1 T	28	1 C	440	10
cornmeal, white or yellow	degermed, enriched	1 T	32	1 C	505	12
cottage cheese, creamed	4% fat small curd	1/4 C	55	1C	230	28
cottage cheese, lowfat	1%	1/4 C	40	1C	165	28
cottage cheese, lowfat	2%	1/4 C	50	1C	200	31
couscous	cooked	1/2 C	90	1 C	175	6

crab	canned	1/4 C	40	1 C	160	28
crab cake	fried	1 oz	45	2 oz	90	11
crab, alaska king	steamed	1 oz	25	4 oz	100	20
crab, blue	steamed	1 oz	30	4 oz	120	25
crab, dungeness	steamed	1 oz	30	4 oz	120	25
crabapple	raw	1 oz	20	1 C sl	85	<.5
cranberries	raw, whole	1/2 C	22	1 C	45	<.5
cranberries	dried, sweetened	1/4 C	90	1/2 C	180	<.5
cranberry sauce	canned, sweetened	1/8 can	85	1/2 C	200	<.5
cream, half and half	fat free	1 T	10	1/4 C	40	1
cream, light	coffee or table	1 T	30	1/4 C	120	3
cream, nondairy topping	whipped, frozen	1 T	15	1/4 C	60	0
cream, sour, lowfat	reduced fat	1 T	20	1/4 C	80	2
cream, sour, nonfat	nonfat	1 T	15	1/4 C	45	2
cream, sour, regular	regular	1 T	25	1/4 C	100	2
cream, whipping	light, unwhipped	1 T	45	1/4 C	180	1
cream, whipping	heavy, unwhipped	1 T	50	1/4 C	200	1
cream, whipping	light, whipped	1 T	10	1/4 C	90	1
cream, whipping	heavy, whipped	1 T	25	1/4 C	100	1
cream, whipping	pressureized	1 T	10	1/4 C	40	<.5
cream cheese	regular	1 T	50	2 T	100	2
cream cheese	regular	1 oz	100	2 oz	200	4
cress	raw & cooked	5 sprigs	3	1 C cook	30	3
cucumber	raw, peeled, sliced	1/2 C	5	1 C	15	1
currants, black	raw	1/2 C	35	1 C	70	2
currants, red or white	raw	1/2 C	30	1 C	65	2

D

dandelion greens	cooked, chopped	1/2 C	20	1 C	35	2

dates, deglet noor	whole, pitted	**1**	25	**4**	100	1
dates, medjool	whole.pitted	**1**	65	**2**	130	1
deer, see venison						
dock (sorrel)	raw, chopped	**1/2 C**	15	**1 C**	30	2
duck	roasted, meat only	**1 oz**	60	**1/2 duck**	445	**52**
duck, wild, breast	raw, meat only	**1 oz**	35	**1/2 brst**	102	**16**

E

egg	large, whole, fresh	**1**	75	**1**	75	**6**
egg white	large	**1**	17	**1**	17	**3.6**
egg yolk	large	**1**	55	**1**	55	**2.7**
egg, duck	whole, fresh	**1**	130	**1**	130	**9**
egg, goose	whole, fresh	**1**	265	**1**	265	**20**
egg, lowfat	large	**1**	70	**1**	70	**6**
egg, quail	whole, fresh	**1**	14	**2**	28	**2**
egg, turkey	whole, fresh	**1**	135	**1**	135	**11**
eggplant	raw	**1 C cubed**	20	**1 whole**	130	6
eggplant	cooked	**1/2 C**	15	**1 C**	35	1
elderberries	raw	**1/2 C**	55	**1 C**	105	1
elk, ground	cooked, patty	**1 oz**	55	**4 oz**	110	**30**
endive	raw, chopped	**1/2 C**	5	**1 C**	10	<.5

F

figs	raw	**1 med**	40	**2 med**	80	1
figs	dried, uncooked	**1 fig**	20	**2**	50	1
filberts or hazelnuts, see nuts						

Fish (for raw, add any cooking oil amount)

fish fillet, battered or breaded	frozen, heated	**1 fillet**	130	**2 fillets**	260	**14**
fish fillet, battered, breaded	fried, fresh	**1 oz**	65	**4 oz**	260	**16**
fish stick	breaded, frozen	**1 stick**	70	**4 sticks**	280	**12**

fish, anchovy, European	canned in oil	**1 oz**	60	**5 anchov**	40	6
fish, bass, mixed species	raw	**1 oz**	30	**4 oz**	120	21
fish, bluefish	raw	**1 oz**	35	**4 oz**	140	23
fish, burbot	raw	**1 oz**	25	**4 oz**	100	22
fish, butterfish	raw	**1 oz**	40	**4 oz**	160	20
fish, carp	raw	**1 oz**	35	**4 oz**	140	20
fish, catfish, channel	raw, farmed	**1 oz**	40	**4 oz**	160	18
fish, catfish, channel	raw, wild	**1 oz**	30	**4 oz**	120	19
fish, cisco	smoked	**1 oz**	50	**2 oz**	100	9
fish, cod, Atlantic, Pacific	raw	**1 oz**	25	**4 oz**	100	20
fish, croaker, Atlantic	raw	**1 oz**	30	**4 oz**	120	20
fish, cusk	raw	**1 oz**	25	**4 oz**	100	22
fish, dolphin fish	raw	**1 oz**	25	**4 oz**	100	21
fish, drum	raw, freshwater	**1 oz**	35	**4 oz**	140	20
fish, eel, mixed species	raw	**1 oz**	50	**4 oz**	200	21
fish, fish portions	frozen, heated	**1 stick**	70	**2x4x1/2**	140	6
fish, flatfish, flounder, sole	raw	**1 oz**	25	**4 oz**	100	21
fish, gefiltefish, commercial	sweet recipe	**1 oz**	25	**1 piece**	35	4
fish, haddock	raw	**1 oz**	25	**4 oz**	100	21
fish, halibut, Atlantic, Pacific	raw	**1 oz**	30	**4 oz**	120	24
fish, herring, Atlantic	raw	**1 oz**	45	**4 oz**	180	20
fish, herring, Atlantic	kippered	**1 oz**	60	**4 fillets**	17	28
fish, herring, Atlantic	pickled	**1 oz**	75	**1 piece**	40	2
fish, herring, Pacific	raw	**1 oz**	55	**4 oz**	220	19
fish, mackerel, Atlantic	raw	**1 oz**	60	**4 oz**	240	21
fish, mackerel, Pacific & Jack	raw	**1 oz**	45	**4 oz**	180	23
fish, mackerel, king	raw	**1 oz**	30	**4 oz**	120	23
fish, mackerel	canned	**1 oz**	50	**1/2 C**	150	22
fish, ocean perch	raw	**1 oz**	25	**4 oz**	100	21

fish, perch, mixed species	raw	**1 oz**	5	**4 oz**	100	22
fish, pike	raw	**1 oz**	25	**4 oz**	100	22
fish, pollock, Atlantic	raw	**1 oz**	25	**4 oz**	100	22
fish, pompano, Florida	raw	**1 oz**	45	**4 oz**	180	21
fish, rockfish, mixed species	raw	**1 oz**	25	**4 oz**	100	21
fish, roughy, orange	raw	**1 oz**	20	**4 oz**	80	19
fish, sable	raw	**1 oz**	55	**2 oz**	110	8
fish, sable	smoked	**1 oz**	75	**2 oz**	150	10
fish, salmon, Atlantic	raw, farmed	**1 oz**	50	**4 oz**	200	23
fish, salmon, coho	raw, wild	**1 oz**	40	**4 oz**	160	24
fish, salmon, chinook	raw, wild	**1 oz**	50	**4 oz**	200	23
fish, salmon, pink	canned	**1 oz**	40	**4 oz**	160	22
fish, salmon, sockeye	canned	**1 oz**	40	**4 oz**	160	23
fish, salmon	smoked	**1 oz**	60	**4 oz**	240	21
fish, sardine, Atlantic	canned in oil	**1 small**	25	**1 can**	190	23
fish, sardine, Pacific	canned/tomato sauce	**1 small**	70	**1 can**	688	77
fish, sea bass, mixed species	raw	**1 oz**	25	**4 oz**	100	21
fish, shad, American	raw	**1 oz**	55	**4 oz**	220	19
fish, shark, mixed species	raw	**1 oz**	35	**4 oz**	140	24
fish, smelt, rainbow	raw	**1 oz**	25	**4 oz**	100	20
fish, snapper, mixed species	raw	**1 oz**	30	**4 oz**	120	23
fish, sturgeon	raw	**1 oz**	30	**4 oz**	120	18
fish, sole or flounder, flatfish	raw	**1 oz**	25	**4 oz**	100	21
fish, swordfish	baked or broiled	**1 oz**	35	**4 oz**	140	22
fish, tilapia	raw	**1 oz**	25	**4 oz**	100	23
fish, trout, mixed species	raw	**1 oz**	40	**4 oz**	160	24
fish, trout	raw, farmed	**1 oz**	40	**4 oz**	160	24
fish, trout	raw, wild	**1 oz**	35	**4 oz**	140	23
fish, tuna, bluefin	raw	**1 oz**	40	**4 oz**	160	26

fish, tuna, yellowfin	raw	**1 oz**	30	**4 oz**	120	**27**
fish, tuna	canned, water pack	**1 oz**	35	**3 oz**	100	**22**
fish, tuna	canned in oil	**1 oz**	55	**3 oz**	170	**25**
fish, turbot, European	raw	**1 oz**	25	**4 oz**	100	**18**
fish, whitefish, mixed species	raw	**1 oz**	40	**4 oz**	160	**22**
fish, whiting	raw	**1 oz**	25	**4 oz**	100	**21**
flour, white	enriched, unbleached	**1 T**	28	**1 C**	455	13
flour, whole wheat	whole grain	**1 T**	25	**1 C**	405	16
french fries S	frozen, heated	**1 oz**	50	**10 fries**	125	2
french fries, steak fries S	frozen, heated	**1 oz**	45	**10 fries**	200	3
fudgesicle bars	fat free	**1 oz**	36	**1 pop**	54	3
fudge bar, Klondike Slim A Bear	98% fat free, no sugar	**1 oz**	35	**1 bar**	92	3
fudgesicle pops	no sugar added	**1 oz**	30	**2 pops**	88	3

G

garlic	raw, cloves	**1 clove**	4	**3**	15	1
garlic	raw, chopped	**1 tsp**	4	**1 T**	15	1
ginger root	fresh, sliced	**1 oz**	15	**1/4 C**	20	<.5
gooseberries	raw	**1/2 C**	30	**1 C**	65	1
grape juice, canned, bottled	unsweetened	**1/2 C**	80	**1 C**	155	1
grapefruit	raw	**1/2 med**	40	**1 med**	80	1
grapefruit juice	canned, unsweetened	**1/2 C**	50	**1 C**	95	1
grapes, seedless	raw	**1/2 C**	55	**1 C**	110	1
grapes, w/seeds	raw	**1/2 C**	50	**1 C**	105	1
green beans, snap, yellow, green	cooked	**1/2 C**	25	**1 C**	45	2
guava	raw, edible portions	**1 fruit**	35	**1 C**	110	4

H

hazelnuts or filberts, see nuts						
honey	raw	**1 tsp**	20	**1 T**	65	<.5

honeydew melon	raw, 6" diameter	**1/4 melon**	115	**1 Ccubes**	60	1
horseradish	prepared	**1 tsp**	2	**1 T**	5	<.5

I

ice cream, chocolate	light, no sugar added	**1/2 C**	110	**1 C**	220	5
ice cream, chocolate	fat free 98%	**1/2 C**	90	**1 C**	180	5
ice cream, chocolate LTN	regular	**1/2 C**	145	**1 C**	290	5
ice cream, chocolate caramel	no sugar added	**1/2 C**	105	**1 C**	215	5
ice cream, chocolate, frozen milk	fat free	**1/2 C**	115	**1 C**	229	6
ice cream, french vanilla LTN	softserve regular	**1/2 C**	190	**1 C**	380	7
ice cream, french vanilla	no sugar added	**1/2 C**	105	**1 C**	210	6
ice cream, vanilla	light	**1/2 C**	125	**1 C**	250	7
ice cream, vanilla LTN	regular	**1/2 C**	145	**1 C**	290	5
ice cream, vanilla	no sugar added	**1/2 C**	100	**1 C**	200	5
ice cream, vanilla fudge twirl	no sugar added	**1/2 C**	110	**1 C**	220	3

J

jam	spread	**1 T**	55	**1 T**	55	<.5
jelly	spread	**1 T**	55	**1 T**	55	<.5

K

kale	cooked	**1/2 C**	20	**1 C**	35	2
kiwi	raw	**1 med**	45	**2 med**	90	2
kohlrabi	cooked, sliced	**1/2 C**	25	**1 C**	50	3
kumquat	raw, edible portions	**1 med**	15	**2 med**	30	1

L

lamb chop	broiled, lean & fat	**1 oz**	90	**4 oz**	360	29
lamb chop	cooked, lean only	**1 oz**	60	**4 oz**	240	34
lamb shoulder	cooked, lean only	**1 oz**	60	**4 oz**	240	28
lamb, leg	raw	**1 oz**	65	**4 oz**	260	20
lamb, leg	cooked	**1 oz**	75	**4 oz**	300	29

leeks	cooked, bulb & lwr leaf	**1/2 C**	10	**1 C**	30	1
lemon	raw	**1/2 med**	10	**1 med**	20	<1
lemon juice	raw or canned	**1 T**	3	**1/4 C**	15	<.5
lentils, see beans						
lettuce, butterhead, Boston	raw, med leaf	**1 leaf**	1	**1 C**	10	1
lettuce, iceburg	raw, med leaf	**1 leaf**	1	**1 C**	10	<.5
lettuce, greenleaf	raw, med leaf	**1 leaf**	1	**1 C**	5	<.5
lettuce, romaine, cos	raw, med leaf	**1 leaf**	1	**1 C**	10	1
lettuce, red leaf	raw, med leaf	**1 leaf**	1	**1 C**	5	<.5
lime	raw	**1/2 small**	10	**1 small**	20	<.5
lime juice	raw, unsweetened	**1 T**	5	**1/4 C**	15	<.5
liquor:gin, vodka, rum, whiskey LTN	80 proof	**1 oz**	65	**1.5 oz**	97	0
liquor:gin, vodka, rum, whiskey LTN	86 proof	**1 oz**	70	**1.5 oz**	105	0
liquor:gin, vodka, rum, whiskey LTN	90 proof	**1 oz**	73	**1.5 oz**	110	0
lobster	steamed	**1 oz**	40	**5 oz**	200	30
loganberries	frozen, thawed	**1/2 C**	40	**1 C**	80	2

M

macadamia nuts, see nuts						
macaroni S	cooked	**1/2 C**	110	**1 C**	220	8
mango	raw, 8 oz	**1 mango**	135	**1 C sl**	105	1
maple syrup	natural	**1 T**	50	**1/4 C**	200	0
margarine	spread	**1 tsp**	35	**1 T**	100	<.5
mayonnaise	fat free	**1 tsp**	5	**1 T**	15	<.5
mayonnaise	light	**1 tsp**	15	**1 T**	50	<.5
mayonnaise	regular	**1 tsp**	35	**1 T**	100	<.5
meatless burger	mix, dry	**1/2 C**	115	**1 C**	230	22
milk, instant, nonfat	dry	**1 T**	15	**1/3 C**	80	8
milk, lowfat	1% fat	**1/2 C**	50	**1C**	100	8

milk, reduced fat	2% fat	1/2 C	60	1C	120	8
milk, skim	nonfat	1/2 C	45	1C	85	8
milk, whole	3.25% fat	1/2 C	70	1C	145	8
molasses	light	1 T	50	1/4 C	200	0
molasses, blackstrap	dark, unrefined	1 T	45	1/4 C	180	0
mushrooms	raw, sliced	1/2 C	10	1 C	20	2
mushrooms	cooked	1/2 C	20	1 C	40	3
mushrooms, shitake	cooked	1/2 C	40	1 C	80	2
mushrooms, shitake	dried	1	10	2	20	1
mustard	yellow	1 tsp	3	1 T	10	1
mustard greens	cooked, chopped	1/2 C	10	1 C	20	3

N

nectarine	raw, 5 oz	1 oz	15	5 oz	75	2
noodles, chow mein S	cooked	1/2 C	120	1 C	235	4
noodles, egg S	cooked	1/2 C	110	1 C	220	7
noodles, egg, spinach S	cooked	1/2 C	105	1 C	210	8
nuts, almonds	raw, whole	1 T	50	1 C	827	30
nuts, almonds	raw, slivered	1 T	40	1 C	624	23
nuts, almonds	raw,sliced	1 T	35	1 C	532	20
nuts, brazil nuts	raw, whole	1 T	55	1 C	918	20
nuts, cashews	dry,oil rstd, w/o salt	1 T	50	1 C	786	21
nuts, filberts or hazelnuts	raw, chopped	1 T	45	1 C	722	17
nuts, filberts or hazelnuts	raw, whole	1 T	55	1 C	848	20
nuts, macadamia	raw	1 T	60	1 C	962	11
nuts, mixed	dry roasted, w/o salt	1 T	50	1 C	814	24
nuts, peanuts	dry roasted, w/o salt	1 T	55	1 C	854	35
nuts, peanuts, spanish	oil roasted, w/o salt	1 T	55	1 C	851	41
nuts, pecans	raw, halves	1 T	40	1 C	684	9

nuts, pecans	raw, chopped	1 T	45	1 C	753	10
nuts, pine nuts	dried	1 T	55	1 C	909	18
nuts, pistachios	raw	1 T	40	1 C	685	25
nuts, walnuts, black	dried, chopped	1 T	50	1 C	772	30
nuts, walnuts, English	raw, halves	1 T	40	1 C	654	15
nuts, walnuts, English	raw, chopped	1 T	45	1 C	765	18
O						
oatmeal, regular	dry, uncooked	1/4 C	75	1/2 C	155	6
oatmeal, regular	cooked	1/2 C	70	1 C	145	6
oils, salad, cooking, vegetable	olive, canola, etc.	1 T	120	1 T	120	<.5
okra	cooked	1/2 C	25	1 C	50	3
olives, black	canned, black	1 lrg	5	10 lrg	50	1
olives, green	canned, green, pickled	1 med	4	10	40	1
onions	raw, chopped	1 T	5	1/2 C	35	1
onions	raw	1 slice	5	1 med	45	1
onions	chopped, sautéed	1/2 C	60	1 C	115	1
onions	dehydrated flakes	1 tsp	5	1 T	20	<.5
onions, green	raw, bulb and tops	1 whole	5	1/2 C	15	1
orange	raw	1 oz	15	4 oz	60	1
orange juice	raw	1/2 C	55	1 C	110	2
orange juice	canned, unsweetened	1/2 C	50	1 C	105	1
orange juice	from frozen concentrate	1/2 C	55	1 C	110	2
oyster, Pacific	raw	1 med	40	4 med	160	5
oyster, eastern	raw, wild	1 med	10	6 med	60	6
oyster, eastern	raw, farmed	1 med	7	6 med	50	4
oyster, eastern	breaded, fried	1 med	30	6 med	175	7
P						
pancakes S	plain, 4" diameter	1	85	2	170	6

pancakes S	whole wheat, 4" diam	**1**	90	**2**	180	8
papaya	raw, edible portion	**1 oz**	10	**1 med**	120	2
parsley	raw, sprigs	**1 T**	1	**10**	4	<.5
parsnips	cooked	**1 oz**	20	**1 C**	110	1
passion fruit (granadilla)	raw, edible portion	**1 oz**	25	**1 fruit**	20	<.5
pasta, various S	cooked	**1/2 C**	100	**1 C**	200	8
peach	raw	**1 oz**	10	**4 oz**	40	1
peach	dried, halves	**1 half**	30	**3**	95	1
peach	canned, juice pack	**1 half**	45	**1 C**	110	2
peanut butter	reg, smooth or chunky	**1 T**	95	**2 T**	190	8
peanuts, see nuts						
pear	raw	**1 oz**	17	**7 oz**	120	1
pear	canned, juice pack	**1 half**	40	**1 C**	125	1
peas	raw	**1/2 C**	60	**1 C**	120	9
peas	canned or frozen	**1/2 C**	60	**1 C**	120	8
peas, edible pod	cooked	**1/2 C**	35	**1 C**	70	5
peas, split, dry	cooked	**1/2 C**	115	**1 C**	230	16
pecans, see nuts						
peppers, hot chili, green, red	raw	**1**	20	**1/2 C**	30	1
peppers, sweet, green, red, yellow	raw	**1 oz**	7	**6 oz**	40	2
pickle relish	sweet	**1 tsp**	7	**1 T**	20	<.5
pickles	dill	**1 slice**	1	**4 slices**	5	1
pickles	sweet (gherkins)	**1 midget**	10	**1/4 C sl**	50	<.5
pickles	sour, slices	**1 slice**	1	**1/4 C**	5	<.5
pimientos	canned	**1 T**	3	**1 med**	15	1
pine nuts, see nuts						
pineapple	raw, diced	**1 oz**	15	**1 C**	75	1
pineapple juice	canned, unsweetened	**1/2 C**	65	**1 C**	130	1
pistachios, see nuts						

pizza, cheese S	12" diameter	**2" slice**	185	**4" sl**	370	varies
pizza, meat/vegetables S	12" diameter	**2" slice**	245	**4" sl**	490	varies
pizza, pepperoni LTN	12" diameter	**2" slice**	240	**4" sl**	480	varies
plums	raw	**1 oz**	15	**2 oz**	30	<.5
pomegranate	raw	**1/2 pom**	50	**1 pom**	105	1
popcorn	plain, air popped	**1 C**	30	**2 C**	60	2
popcorn	popped w/oil, salted	**1 C**	55	**2 C**	110	2
pork, bacon LTN	pan fried	**1 oz**	150	**1 slice**	40	3
pork, bacon, Canadian style LTN	unheated	**1 oz**	45	**2 sl**	90	12
pork, bacon, Canadian style LTN	cooked	**1 oz**	50	**2 sl**	90	12
pork, chop	pan broiled, lean	**1 oz**	50	**4 oz**	200	33

pork, ham   (All ham is LTN due to processing and curing, but some lean may be tolerated.)

pork, ham	cured, roasted, lean	**1 oz**	60	**4 oz**	240	35
pork, ham	cured, rstd, lean & fat	**1 oz**	75	**4 oz**	310	31
pork, ham, extra lean	cured, roasted	**1 oz**	40	**4 oz**	160	24
pork, ham, extra lean	cured, unheated	**1 oz**	35	**4 oz**	140	22
pork, ham, extra lean & regular	cured, unheated	**1 oz**	45	**4 oz**	180	21
pork, ham, lean & fat	cured, unheated	**1 oz**	70	**4 oz**	280	21
pork, ham, rump half	fresh, roasted, lean	**1 oz**	60	**4 oz**	240	35
pork, ham, shank half	fresh, roasted, lean	**1 oz**	60	**4 oz**	240	32
pork, ham, whole	cured, unheated	**1 oz**	40	**4 oz**	160	25
pork, ham, whole, lean only	cured, roasted	**1 oz**	45	**4 oz**	180	28
pork, loin roast	cooked, lean only	**1 oz**	65	**4 oz**	260	31
pork, ribs, country style	cooked, lean & fat	**1 oz**	85	**4 oz**	340	27
pork, ribs, country style	cooked, lean only	**1 oz**	65	**4 oz**	260	30
pork, sausage, ground LTN	patty, cooked	**1 oz**	100	**2 oz**	200	10
pork, sausage, link LTN	cooked	**1 link**	80	**2 links**	160	14
pork, shoulder, roast	cooked, lean	**1 oz**	65	**4 oz**	260	27
pork, shoulder, steak	cooked, lean	**1 oz**	90	**4 oz**	320	33

pork, spareribs	cooked, lean & fat	**1 oz**	110	**4 oz**	440	**33**
pork, tenderloin	cooked, lean	**1 oz**	55	**4 oz**	220	**34**
potato	baked, flesh only	**1 oz**	26	**10 oz**	260	6
potato	raw, diced or sliced	**1/2 C**	60	**1 C**	120	3
potato	mashed w/milk & butter	**1/2 C**	110	**1 C**	220	4
potato	boiled, peeled	**1/2 C**	65	**1 C**	135	3
potato, french fries, fast food LTN	french fries	**1 oz**	100	**3 oz**	300	2
potato, wedges	from frozen	**1 oz**	35	**10 oz**	350	6
potato chips LTN	plain	**1 oz**	150	**6 oz**	900	12
prune juice	canned	**1/2 C**	90	**1 C**	180	2
prunes	dried	**1 prune**	20	**5**	100	1
pudding, instant, dry (add milk)	fat free, sugar free	**1 oz**	95	**8 g pkt**	25	<.5
pudding, instant, chocolate	prepared w/2% milk	**1/2 C**	155	**1 C**	310	9
pumpkin	canned	**1/2 C**	40	**1 C**	85	3
pumpkin and squash seed kernels	dried	**1 T**	45	**1 C**	720	39
pumpkin and squash seed kernels	roasted, w/o salt	**1 T**	42	**1 C**	680	35
pumpkin and squash seeds	whole, rstd, w/o salt	**1 T**	20	**1 C**	285	12

Q, R

radish	raw	**1 radish**	1	**10**	10	<.5
raisins	seedless	**1 T**	30	**1/4 C**	120	1
raspberries	raw	**1/2 C**	30	**1 C**	65	2
raspberries	frozen, sweetened	**1 T**	15	**1/4 C**	85	<.5
rice, brown, medium/long grain	cooked	**1/2 C**	105	**1 C**	215	4
rice, white, long grain	cooked	**1/2 C**	100	**1 C**	205	4
rice, white, short/medium grain	cooked	**1/2 C**	120	**1 C**	210	4
rice, wild	cooked	**1/4 C**	40	**1/2 C**	80	3
rice cakes, brown rice	plain	**1 oz**	110	**1 cake**	35	1
rice cakes, brown rice	sesame seed	**1 oz**	111	**1 cake**	35	1

rutabaga	cooked, diced	1/2 C	30	1 C	65	2
S						
salad dressings	lowfat	1 T	20	1 T	20	<.5
salad dressings	regular	1 T	70	1 T	70	<.5
salsa	ready to serve	1 T	5	1/4 C	20	<.5
sauerkraut	canned, undrained	1/2 C	20	1 C	45	2
scallop	raw	1 oz	25	4 oz	100	20
scallop	breaded, fried	1 oz	60	2 lrg	70	6
sesame seeds	whole, dried	1 T	50	1 C	825	26
shallots	raw, chopped	1 T	7	1/4 C	30	1
shrimp	fresh	1 oz	30	4 lrg	30	6
shrimp	breaded, fried	1 oz	70	3 oz	210	18
shrimp	breaded, fried	1 large	75	6 lrg	450	38
soda pop, regular LTN	cola, root beer, etc	1 oz	12	12 oz	135-180	0
soda pop, diet	cola, root beer, etc	1 oz	0	12 oz	0 - 5	0
soda, club	carbonated, plain	1 oz	0	12 oz	0	0
sour cream	reduced fat, cultured	1 T	20	1/4 C	80	2
sour cream	nonfat	1 T	10	1/4 C	40	2
sour cream	regular	1 T	25	1/4 C	100	3
soy burger	mix, dry	1/2 C	115	1 C	230	22
soy sauce and tamari	regular	1 tsp	3	1 T	10	1
spaghetti S	enriched, cooked	1/2 C	110	1 C	220	8
spaghetti, spinach S	cooked	1/2 C	90	1 C	180	6
spaghetti, whole wheat S	cooked	1/2 C	85	1 C	175	7
spaghetti sauce	ready to serve	1/2 C	90	1 C	185	5
spinach	raw	1 leaf	2	1 C	10	1
spinach	cooked	1/2 C	20	1 C	40	5
squash, summer, all varieties	cooked, sliced	1/2 C	20	1 C	35	2

squash, winter, all varieties	cooked, baked	1/2 C	40	1 C	75	2
strawberries	raw, sliced	1/2 C	25	1 C	50	1
strawberries	frozen, unsweetened	1/4 C	25	1/2 C	50	1
submarine sandwich S	tuna salad w/mayo	1 oz	65	8 oz	585	30
submarine sandwich S	turkey, ham, vegetables	1 oz	55	8 oz	456	22
submarine sandwich S	roast beef	1 oz	55	8 oz	410	29
sugar, brown	refined	1 tsp	10	1 T	35	0
sugar, raw brown	unrefined	1 tsp	5	1 T	15	<.5
sugar, white granulated LTN	beet or cane, refined	1 tsp	15	1 T	45	0
sunflower seed kernels	dried	1 T	50	1 C	821	33
sunflower seed kernels	dry roasted, w/o salt	1 T	45	1 C	745	25
sunflower seeds w/hulls	dried	1 T	15	1 C	262	10
sweet potato	baked, boiled	1 oz	25	10 oz	250	6
Swiss chard	cooked, chopped	1/2 C	15	1 C	35	3
syrup, maple	natural maple	1 T	50	1/4 C	200	0

T

tangerine	raw	1 oz	15	4 oz	60	1
tea	black, herb	1 oz	0	1 C	2	0
tofu	firm	1 oz	20	2 oz	40	4
tofu	soft	1 oz	15	2 oz	30	4
tomato	raw	1/4" sl	5	1 C	30	2
tomato	stewed	1/2 C	40	1 C	80	2
tomato juice	canned	1/2 C	20	1 C	40	2
tomato paste	canned	1/2 C	105	6 oz can	140	7
tomato puree	canned	1/2 C	50	1 C	100	4
tomato sauce	canned	1/2 C	40	1 C	80	3
tomato, chopped or sliced	raw	1/2 C	15	1 C	30	2
tortilla, yellow corn S	6" diameter	1	60	2	180	2

tortilla, flour S	7 to 8" diameter	**1**	145	**2**	290	8
turkey, dark meat	roasted, mcat only	**1 oz**	55	**4 oz**	220	32
turkey, light meat	roasted, meat only	**1 oz**	45	**4 oz**	180	34
turnip	cooked, cubes	**1/2 C**	15	**1 C**	35	1
turnip greens	cooked	**1/2 C**	15	**1 C**	30	2

U, V, W

vegetable juice	canned	**1/2 C**	25	**1 C**	45	1
vegetable stew meatless	homemade	**1 C**	60	**2 C**	120	4
vegi burger	cooked	**1 oz**	30	**3 oz**	90	14
vinegar	cider, distilled	**1 T**	2	**1/4 C**	10	0
venison	cooked	**1 oz**	45	**4 oz**	180	34
venison, ground	cooked, patty	**1 oz**	55	**4 oz**	110	30
venison, loin steak	cooked	**1 oz**	45	**4 oz**	180	34
walnuts, see nuts						
water chestnuts, Chinese	canned	**4 avg**	15	**1 C sl**	35	1
watercress	raw, sprigs	**10**	3	**1 C**	5	1
watermelon	raw, cubed	**1 oz**	10	**1 C**	45	1
wheat bran	raw	**1 T**	8	**1 C**	120	9
wheat germ	raw	**1 T**	25	**2 T**	50	4
wheat germ oil	supplement/Vit E	**1 tsp**	40	**1 T**	125	<.5
whipped topping	frozen	**1 T**	15	**1/4 C**	60	0
whipped topping, light	frozen	**1 T**	10	**1/4 C**	40	0
whole wheat natural cereal	dry, uncooked	**1/4 C**	80	**1/2 C**	160	5
whole wheat natural cereal	cooked	**1/2 C**	160	**1 C**	160	5
wine, dessert	sweet	**1 oz**	45	**4 oz**	180	<.5
wine, table	red, white	**1 oz**	25	**6 oz**	150	<.5

X, Y, Z

yams	baked, boiled	**1 oz**	35	**10 oz**	350	4

yogurt butter	oil/yogurt spread	**1 tsp**	15	**1 T**	45	0
yogurt, frozen, soft serve LTN	choc, vanilla	**1/2 C**	115	**1 C**	230	6
yogurt, frozen, chocolate, nonfat	no sugar added	**1/2 C**	100	**1 C**	199	8
yogurt, lowfat	artificial sweetener	**1 oz**	14	**8 oz**	110	8
yogurt, lowfat LTN	sugar, fruit ,flavorings	**1 oz**	29	**8 oz**	240	11
yogurt, lowfat	all natural, plain	**1 oz**	19	**8 oz**	150	11
yogurt, lowfat plus milk solids	plain	**1 oz**	18	**8 oz**	145	12
yogurt, nonfat	artificial sweetener	**1 oz**	13	**8 oz**	100	9
yogurt, nonfat	plain	**1 oz**	16	**8 oz**	130	13
yogurt, nonfat LTN	sugar, fruit, flavorings	**1 oz**	27	**8 oz**	215	10
yogurt, whole	plain	**1 oz**	18	**8 oz**	140	8

Love Your Diet
Calorie Counter

Foods Not to Eat

FAST FOODS & LTN FOODS

Food	A Amt	Calories	B Amt	Calories	B Protein grams EAA
A B					
biscuit, scone	**1 oz**	100	**3 oz**	300	4
biscuit, w/bacon, egg, & cheese, McDonald's	**1 oz**	86	**1**	441	19
biscuit, w/egg	**1 oz**	78	**1**	373	12
biscuit, w/egg & bacon	**1 oz**	86	**1**	458	17
biscuit, w/egg & ham	**1 oz**	68	**1**	461	20
biscuit, w/egg & sausage	**1 oz**	92	**1**	581	19
biscuit, w/egg & steak	**1 oz**	79	**1**	410	18
biscuit, w/ham	**1 oz**	97	**1**	386	13
biscuit, w/sausage	**1 oz**	111	**1**	485	12
bologna, beef	**1 oz**	89	**28g sl**	88	3
bologna, beef & pork	**1 oz**	87	**1 oz sl**	87	4
bologna, beef & pork, low fat	**1 oz**	65	**28g sl**	64	3
bologna, chicken, pork	**1 oz**	95	**28g sl**	94	3
bologna, chicken, pork, beef	**1 oz**	77	**28g sl**	76	3
bologna, pork	**1 oz**	70	**28g sl**	69	4
bologna, turkey	**1 oz**	59	**28g sl**	59	3
bread, mixed grain, shelf, sliced	**1 oz**	71	**26g sl**	65	3
bread, white, shelf, sliced	**1 oz**	75	**25g sl**	66	2
bread, whole wheat, shelf, sliced	**1 oz**	70	**28g sl**	69	3
Breakfast, McDonald's Big	**1 oz**	78	**1**	732	28
Breakfast, McDonald's Deluxe	**1 oz**	79	**1**	1219	33
Burrito Supreme, w/beef, Taco Bell	**1 oz**	54	**1**	469	20
Burrito Supreme, w/chicken, Taco Bell	**1 oz**	51	**1**	444	24
Burrito Supreme, w/steak, Taco Bell	**1 oz**	52	**1**	454	23
burrito, bean, Taco Bell	**1 oz**	58	**1**	404	16

burrito, w/beans	**1 oz**	58	**2 pieces**	447	14
burrito, w/beans & cheese	**1 oz**	58	**2 pieces**	378	**15**
burrito, w/beans, cheese, & beef	**1 oz**	46	**2 pieces**	331	**15**
burrito, w/beef	**1 oz**	67	**2 pieces**	524	**27**

C

cake, angel food	**1 oz**	73	**3 oz**	219	5
cake, boston cream pie	**1 oz**	71	**1/6 pie**	232	2
cake, brownie	**1 oz**	132	**2" sq**	112	2
cake, chocolate w/frosting	**1 oz**	104	**1/8 cake**	235	3
cake, fruitcake	**1 oz**	92	**2 oz**	185	2
cake, gingerbread	**1 oz**	101	**1/9 piece**	263	3
cake, pineapple upside-down	**1 oz**	90	**4 oz**	367	4
cake, pound prepared w/butter	**1 oz**	110	**2 oz**	232	3
cake, snack cake, sponge, crème-filled	**1 oz**	103	**1 cake**	157	1
cake, snack cupcakes, choc w/frosting, crème-filled	**1 oz**	107	**1 ccake**	188	2
cake, sponge	**1 oz**	82	**2 oz**	164	3
cake, white, w/coconut frosting	**1 oz**	101	**2 oz**	202	2
cake, yellow, w/vanilla frosting	**1 oz**	106	**2 oz**	112	2
candy, 5th Avenue candy bar	**1 oz**	137	**2 oz**	270	5
candy, Almond Joy	**1 oz**	136	**1.8g pkg**	235	2
candy, average	**1 oz**	135	**2 oz**	270	2
candy, Caramello candy bar	**1 oz**	131	**1.6 oz bar**	208	3
candy, fudge, chocolate w/nuts, from recipe	**1 oz**	131	**2 oz**	262	2
candy, fudge, chocolate, prepared from recipe	**1 oz**	117	**2 oz**	234	1
candy, fudge, vanilla, prepared from recipe	**1 oz**	109	**2 oz**	218	<1
candy, M&M Mars, TWIX choc fudge cookie bars	**1 oz**	156	**2 oz bar**	312	4
candy, milk chocolate bar	**1 oz**	152	**1.5 oz bar**	235	2
candy, Milky Way candy bar	**1 oz**	124	**3.6 oz bar**	450	2

candy, Mounds	**1 oz**	138	**1.9 oz bar**	258	2
candy, Reese's Peanut Butter Cups	**1 oz**	146	**2 cups**	232	3
cereal, bran flakes	**1 oz**	91	**1 C**	128	4
cereal, composite character (movies, TV)	**1 oz**	110	**1 C**		
cereal, corn flakes	**1 oz**	102	**1 C**	101	2
cereal, corn grits, instant, dry	**1 oz**	97	**1 pkt**	96	2
cereal, General Mills Cheerios	**1 oz**	105	**1 C**	111	4
cereal, General Mills Frosted Cheerios	**1 oz**	108	**1 C**	115	2
cereal, General Mills Lucky Charms	**1 oz**	108	**1 C**	114	2
cereal, General Mills Wheat Chex	**1 oz**	98	**1 C**	104	3
cereal, General Mills Wheaties	**1 oz**	101	**1 C**	106	3
cereal, Kellogg's Cocoa Krispies	**1 oz**	108	**1 C**	157	2
cereal, Kellogg's Frosted Flakes	**1 oz**	104	**1 C**	152	1
cereal, Kellogg's Frosted Flakes, 1/3 less sugar	**1 oz**	107	**1 C**	117	2
cereal, Kellogg's Product 19	**1 oz**	94	**1 C**	100	2
cereal, Kellogg's Rice Krispies	**1 oz**	110	**1 C**	108	2
cereal, Kellogg's Special K	**1 oz**	107	**1 C**	117	7
cereal, Kraft, Post, corn flakes, Post Toasties	**1 oz**	102	**1 C**	101	2
cereal, Kraft, Post, frosted shredded wht, bite-size,	**1 oz**	100	**1 C**	183	4
cereal, Kraft, Post, Marshmallow Alpha-bits	**1 oz**	113	**1 C**	115	2
cereal, Kraft, Post, Raisin Bran	**1 oz**	90	**1 C**	178	5
cereal, Kraft, Post, shredded wheat, spoon size	**1 oz**	96	**1 C**	167	5
cereal, oats, instant, fortified, plain, dry	**1 oz**	105	**1 pkt**	103	4
cereal, puffed rice	**1 oz**	109	**1 C**	54	1
cereal, puffed wheat	**1 oz**	104	**1 C**	44	2
cereal, Quaker Cap'n Crunch	**1 oz**	114	**1 C**	144	2
cereal, Quaker Oats and Honey	**1 oz**	129	**1/2 C**	232	5
cereal, Quaker Oats Life	**1 oz**	106	**1 C**	160	4

cereal, Ralston Crispy Rice	1 oz	103	1 C	102	2
cereal, shredded wheat, plain, biscuit	1	84	2	155	5
cheeseburger, Burger King	1 oz	81	1	380	19
cheeseburger, large, double patty, w/cond & veg	1 oz	77	1	704	38
cheeseburger, large, single patty, w/bacon & cond	1 oz	88	1	608	32
cheeseburger, large, single patty, w/cond & veg.	1 oz	73	1	563	28
cheeseburger, McDonald's	1 oz	75	1	313	15
cheeseburger, McDonald's double	1 oz	75	1	458	26
cheeseburger, regular, double patty w/cond & veg	1 oz	71	1	417	21
cheeseburger, triple patty, plain	1 oz	74	1	796	56
cheeseburger, Wendy's Classic Single w/cheese	1 oz	63	1	522	35
chicken, boneless, breaded, fried	1 oz	84	6 pieces	285	15
chicken, breaded, fried, dark meat	1 oz	82	2 pieces	431	30
chicken, breaded, fried, light meat	1 oz	86	2 pieces	494	36
chicken, Burger King Chicken Tenders	1 oz	82	6 pieces	266	13
chicken, Burger King Chicken Whopper sandwich	1 oz	61	1	588	32
chicken, Burger King Original Chicken sandwich	1 oz	81	1	583	31
chicken, fillet sandwich	1 oz	80	1	515	24
chicken, fillet sandwich w/cheese	1 oz	79	1	632	29
chicken, McDonald's Caesar Salad w/crispy chicken	1 oz	27	1 salad	294	25
chicken, McDonald's Chicken McGrill w/mayo	1 oz	54	1	405	28
chicken, McDonald's Chicken McGrill w/o mayo	1 oz	43	1	298	28
chicken, McDonald's Crispy Chicken sand w/mayo	1 oz	65	1	504	24
chicken, McDonald's Crispy Chicken sand w/o mayo	1 oz	55	1	398	24
chicken, McDonald's McNuggets	1 oz	75	6 pieces	253	15
chicken, Taco Bell Burrito Supreme w/chicken	1 oz	51	1	444	24
chicken, Taco Bell soft taco w/chicken	1 oz	57	1	200	14
chicken, Wendy's Chicken Nuggets	1 oz	95	5 pieces	250	12

chicken, Wendy's Homestyle Chicken Fillet Sand	**1 oz**	61	**1**	492	**32**
chicken, Wendy's Ultimate Chicken Grill Sandwich	**1 oz**	51	**1**	403	**33**
chips, cheese flavored puffs or twists, corn based	**1 oz**	158	**6 oz**	948	10
chips, cheese flvrd puffs or twists, corn based, lowfat	**1 oz**	122	**6 oz**	732	14
chips, corn based, extruded, barbecue flavor	**1 oz**	148	**6 oz**	888	12
chips, corn based, extruded, plain	**1 oz**	147	**6 oz**	882	10
chips, potato, barbecue flavor	**1 oz**	139	**6 oz**	834	13
chips, potato, plain, salted	**1 oz**	155	**6 oz**	931	11
chips, potato, reduced fat	**1 oz**	134	**6 oz**	804	12
chips, potato, reduced fat, no salt	**1 oz**	138	**6 oz**	828	12
chips, potato, restructured, baked	**1 oz**	133	**6 oz**	798	9
chips, potato, sour cream & onion flavor	**1 oz**	151	**6 oz**	906	14
chips, taco, plain	**1 oz**	141	**6 oz**	846	13
chips, tortilla, lowfat, unsalted	**1 oz**	118	**6 oz**	708	19
chips, tortilla, nacho flavor	**1 oz**	144	**6 oz**	864	14
chips, tortilla, nacho flavor, reduced fat	**1 oz**	126	**6 oz**	756	15
chips, tortilla, taco flavor	**1 oz**	136	**6 oz**	816	13
chips, tortilla, white corn, plain	**1 oz**	138	**6 oz**	828	13
cinnamon roll, McDonald's, warm	**1 oz**	113	**3.7 oz**	418	8
cinnamon roll, McDonald's, warm deluxe	**1 oz**	104	**5.7 oz**	595	9
cinnamon roll, or sweet roll, w/raisins, commercial	**1 oz**	105	**83 g**	309	5
cinnamon roll, refrigerated dough, w/frosting	**1 oz**	94	**30 g**	100	2
cookies, brownies, commercially prepared	**1 oz**	115	**2 3/4"sq**	227	3
cookies, butter	**1 oz**	132	**5g cke**	23	<.5
cookies, chocolate chip, fast foods	**1 oz**	120	**55g box**	233	3
cookies, chocolate chip, McDonald's	**1 oz**	136	**2 oz cke**	269	3
cookies, chocolate chip, regular	**1 oz**	139	**14g cke**	68	1
cookies, chocolate, sandwich, crème filling	**1 oz**	132	**10g cke**	47	1

cookies, chocolate, sandwich, crème filling, dietary	**1 oz**	131	**10g cke**	46	<.5
cookies, chocolate, sandwich, extra crème filling	**1 oz**	141	**13g cke**	65	1
cookies, coconut macaroons	**1 oz**	115	**24g cke**	97	1
cookies, fig bars	**1 oz**	99	**16g cke**	56	1
cookies, ginger snaps	**1 oz**	118	**7g cke**	29	2
cookies, graham crackers, plain, honey, cinnamon	**1 oz**	120	**4 sq crkr**	59	1
cookies, lady fingers	**1 oz**	103	**11g cke**	40	1
cookies, marshmallow pie, chocolate coated	**1 oz**	119	**39g pie**	164	2
cookies, molasses	**1 oz**	122	**32g cke**	138	2
cookies, oatmeal, regular	**1 oz**	128	**18g cke**	81	1
cookies, peanut butter, regular	**1 oz**	135	**15g cke**	72	1
cookies, shortbread, plain	**1 oz**	142	**8g cke**	40	<.5
cookies, sugar wafers, w/crème filling	**1 oz**	145	**9g wafer**	46	<.5
cookies, sugar, regular	**1 oz**	136	**15g cke**	72	1
cookies, vanilla sandwich, w/crème filling	**1 oz**	237	**10g cke**	48	<.5
cookies, vanilla wafers	**1 oz**	125	**4g cke**	18	<.5
crackers, cheese, regular	**1 oz**	143	**1" sq**	5	<.5
crackers, cheese, sandwich-type, cheese filling	**1 oz**	139	**1sndwch**	32	<1
crackers, cheese, sandwich-type, peanut btr filling	**1 oz**	141	**1 sndwch**	32	1
crackers, graham, plain, honey, cinnamon	**1 oz**	120	**4 sq crkr**	59	1
crackers, matzo, plain	**1 oz**	112	**28g crkr**	111	3
crackers, melba toast, plain	**1 oz**	111	**5g piece**	20	1
crackers, rye, crispbread	**1 oz**	104	**10g crkr**	37	1
crackers, rye, wafers, plain	**1 oz**	95	**11g crkr**	37	1
crackers, saltine (includes oyster, soda, soup)	**1 oz**	121	**6g crkr**	26	1
crackers, standard, snack-type, regular	**1 oz**	142	**4g crkr**	20	<.5
crackers, standard, snack-type, w/cheese filling	**1 oz**	135	**7g crkr**	33	1
crackers, sandard, snack-type, w/ peanut butter fill	**1 oz**	140	**7g crkr**	35	1

crackers, wheat, regular	1 oz	134	2g crkr	9	<.5
crackers, whole wheat	1 oz	126	4g crkr	18	1
croissant, w/egg & cheese	1 oz	82	1	368	13
croissant, w/egg, cheese, & bacon	1 oz	91	1	413	16
croissant, w/egg, cheese, & ham	1 oz	88	1	474	19
croissant, w/egg, cheese, & sausage	1 oz	93	1	523	20

D

danish pastry, cheese	1 oz	110	91 g	353	6
danish pastry, cinnamon	1 oz	113	88 g	349	5
danish pastry, fruit	1 oz	101	94 g	334	5
Deluxe Breakfast, McDonald's	1 oz	79	1	1219	33
doughnuts, cake, chocolate, glazed	1 oz	116	3 3/4"d	250	3
doughnuts, cake-type, plain	1 oz	119	3 1/4"d	198	2
doughnuts, cake-type, sugared or glazed	1 oz	121	3" diam	192	2
doughnuts, raised, glazed, yeast-leavened	1 oz	114	2 oz med	228	4
doughnuts, yeast-leavened, crème filling	1 oz	102	3 oz oval	306	5
doughnuts, yeast-leavened, jelly filling	1 oz	96	3 oz	288	5

E

éclair, custard filled w/chocolate glaze (&crème puff)	1 oz	74	3 oz	222	5
egg & cheese sandwich	1 oz	66	1	340	16
Egg & Sausage McMuffin, McDonald's	1 oz	77	1	446	21
Egg McMuffin, McDonald's	1 oz	60	1	290	18
egg, ham, & cheese sandwich	1 oz	69	1	347	20
eggs scrambled, McDonald's	1 oz	52	2 eggs	184	15

F

fish fillet sandwich w/tartar sauce	1 oz	77	1	431	21
fish fillet sandwich w/tartar sauce & cheese	1 oz	81	1	523	21
frankfurter, beef	1 oz	94	1 57g	188	6

frankfurter, beef & pork, low fat	1 oz	44	1 57g	88	6
frankfurter, chicken	1 oz	64	1 45g	102	6
frankfurter, meat	1 oz	82	1 52g	151	5
frankfurter, meatless	1 oz	66	1 70g	163	14
frankfurter, Oscar Mayer wieners, beef	1 oz	93	1 45g	147	5
frankfurter, Oscar Mayer wieners, beef, fat free	1 oz	22	1 50g	39	7
frankfurter, Oscar Mayer wieners, pork, turkey, beef	1 oz	55	1 57g	111	7
frankfurter, pork	1 oz	76	76g link	204	10
french fries, Burger King, king size	1 oz	94	1	642	7
french fries, Burger King, large	1 oz	94	1	530	6
french fries, Burger King, medium	1 oz	94	1	387	4
french fries, Burger King, small	1 oz	94	1	245	3
french fries, McDonald's, large	1 oz	87	1	522	6
french fries, McDonald's, medium	1 oz	87	1	350	4
french fries, McDonald's, small	1 oz	87	1	227	3
french fries, Wendy's, biggie	1 oz	90	1	507	6
french fries, Wendy's, great biggie	1 oz	90	1	606	7
french fries, Wendy's, medium	1 oz	90	1	453	6
french toast, w/butter	1 oz	75	2 slices	356	10
frozen novelties, vanilla ice cream w/choc coating	1 oz	94	1 bar	166	2

G

gravy, beef, canned	1/4 C	30	1 C	123	6
gravy, chicken, canned	1/4 C	47	1 C	188	5
gravy, turkey, canned	1/4 C	30	1 C	121	6

H

ham & cheese sandwich	1 oz	68	1	352	21
hamburger, Burger King	1 oz	78	1	333	17
hamburger, large, double patty, w/condiments & veg	1 oz	68	1	540	34

hamburger, large, single patty, w/condiments	1 oz	70	1	427	23
hamburger, McDonald's	1 oz	71	1	265	13
hamburger, regular, double patty, w/condiments	1 oz	76	1	576	32
hamburger, regular, single patty, plain	1 oz	86	1	274	12
hamburger, regular, single patty, w/condiments	1 oz	73	1	272	12
hamburger, regular, single patty, w/cond & veg	1 oz	72	1	279	13
hamburger, regular, triple patty, w/condiments	1 oz	76	1	692	50
hamburger, Wendy's Classic single hamburger	1 oz	60	1	464	28
hash browns, McDonald's	1 oz	73	1	136	1

I J K L M

liverwurst, pork	1 oz	92	16g sl	59	3

N

Nachos Supreme, Taco Bell	1 oz	70	1 195g	480	15
Nachos, Taco Bell	1 oz	104	1 99g	362	5

O

onion rings, breaded & fried	1 oz	94	8 to 9	276	4

P

pancakes, w/butter & syrup	1 oz	64	2 cakes	520	8
pickle & pimiento loaf	1 oz	64	38g sl	86	4
pie, apple, commercially prepared	1 oz	67	4 oz	268	2
pie, blueberry, commercially prepared	1 oz	66	4 oz	264	2
pie, cherry, commercially prepared	1 oz	74	4 oz	296	2
pie, chocolate crème, commercially prepared	1 oz	86	4 oz	344	3
pie, coconut crème, commercially prepared	1 oz	84	4 oz	336	2
pie, crust, standard type, from recipe, baked	1 oz	149	9" whole	949	12
pie, fried pie, fruit	1 oz	90	5"x3 3/4"	404	4
pie, fried pie, lemon	1 oz	90	5"x3 3/4"	404	4

pie, McDonald's baked apple pie	**1 oz**	92	**1 pie**	249	2
pie, pecan, commercially prepared	**1 oz**	113	**4 oz**	452	5
pie, pumpkin, commercially prepared	**1 oz**	60	**4 oz**	240	4
pizza, 14", cheese, regular crust	**1 oz**	75	**1 whole**	2389	108
pizza, 14", cheese, thick crust	**1 oz**	77	**1 whole**	2655	117
pizza, 14", cheese, thin crust	**1 oz**	86	**1 whole**	1906	89
pizza, 14", meat & vegetable, regular crust	**1 oz**	69	**1 whole**	2850	129
pizza, 14", pepperoni, regular crust	**1 oz**	78	**1 whole**	2647	118
pizza, 14", pepperoni, thick crust	**1 oz**	81	**1 whole**	2826	124
potato wedges, from frozen	**1 oz**	35	**10 oz**	350	6
pudding, instant, chocolate, prepared w/2% milk	**1/2 C**	155	**1 C**	310	9
pudding, instant, chocolate, prepared w/whole milk	**1/2 C**	326	**1 C**	652	9

Q R S

salami, cooked, beef	**1 oz**	73	**26g sl**	67	3
salami, cooked, beef & pork	**1 oz**	71	**23g sl**	58	3
salami, dry or hard, pork	**1 oz**	115	**10g sl**	41	2
sausage, beef, cured, smoked	**1 oz**	88	**43g saus**	134	6
sausage, Italian, pork, cooked	**1 oz**	98	**83g link**	286	16
sausage, Polish, pork	**1 oz**	92	**227g**	740	32
sausage, thuringer, summer, beef & pork	**1 oz**	103	**56g sl**	203	10
shake, chocolate, McDonald's, triple thick, large	**1 oz**	46	**1 32 oz**	1162	26
shake, chocolate, McDonald's, triple thick, medium	**1 oz**	46	**1 21 oz**	771	17
shake, chocolate, McDonald's, triple thick, small	**1 oz**	46	**1 16 oz**	580	13
shake, strawberry, McDonald's, triple thick, large	**1 oz**	45	**1 32 oz**	1119	25
shake, strawberry, McDonald's, triple thick, medium	**1 oz**	45	**1 21 oz**	741	16
shake, strawberry, McDonald's, triple thick, small	**1 oz**	45	**1 16 oz**	559	12
shake, vanilla, Burger King, medium	**1 oz**	42	**1 16 oz**	667	13
shake, vanilla, Burger King, small	**1 oz**	42	**1 12 oz**	501	10

shake, vanilla, McDonald's, triple thick, large	**1 oz**	35	**1 32 oz**	1104	**25**
shake, vanilla, McDonald's, triple thick, medium	**1 oz**	35	**1 21 oz**	733	**16**
shake, vanilla, McDonald's, triple thick, small	**1 oz**	35	**1 16 oz**	552	**12**

T - Z

taco salad	**1 oz**	40	**1.5 C**	279	13
taco salad, Taco Bell	**1 oz**	48	**1 533g**	906	**35**
taco, large	**1 oz**	61	**1 263g**	568	**32**
taco, original, w/beef, Taco Bell	**1 oz**	67	**1 78g**	184	**8**
taco, small	**1 oz**	61	**1 171g**	369	**21**
taco, soft, w/beef, Taco Bell	**1 oz**	62	**1 99g**	217	**12**
taco, soft, w/chicken, Taco Bell	**1 oz**	57	**1 99g**	200	**14**
taco, soft, w/steak, Taco Bell	**1 oz**	64	**1 127g**	286	**15**